Paleo for Beginners

The Simple Step by Step Paleo Diet Plan for Beginners Including Recipes and Custom Meal Plans

by Jennifer Roberts

Paleo for Beginners

XMS Publishing
1391 NW St. Lucie West Blvd
Suite 247
Port St Lucie, FL 34986

First Published, 2013

ISBN-13: 978-0615843346

ISBN-10: 0615843344

Published in the United States of America

Customer Only Bonus

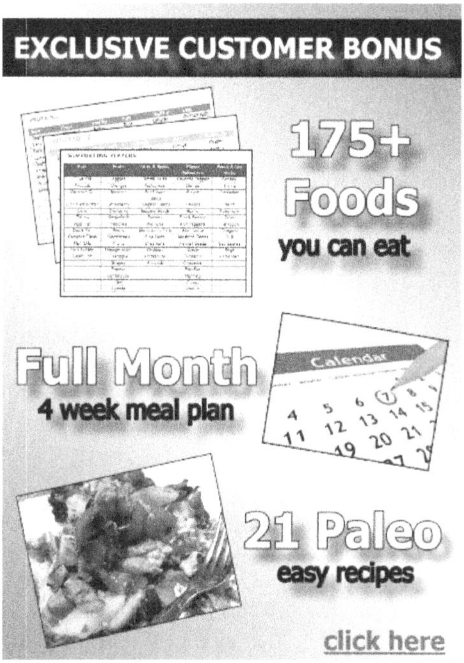

You can also get the customer appreciation bonus here:

http://just4u.co/o/paleobonus

Contents

Introduction

If you turn on the television or see the news these days obesity is on the rise in a major way. Not just in the U.S., but it is a global issue affecting main different countries. As things have become more fast paces everyone is looking for short cuts and with short cuts comes possible issues. The food that we consume is not what our bodies need to be healthy. Let's dispel one thing right in the beginning here. This is not about counting calories, but returning to a natural diet that our body needs to thrive.

It is not about counting calories.

The foundation of the Paleo diet is driven from the philosophy and proven fact about how people ate 10,000 years ago. There was not fast food and processed packages for quick consumption. People had to actually get their food naturally from the earth. The great thing is that there was not widespread disease and the other multitude of health programs that a lot of people suffer from. Things like cardiovascular complications, cancer, and even arthritis. This is what makes this meal plan one that you can easy check. All you have to do it ask yourself:

Would a caveman eat this?

Back in the day the human body was wired and programmed to protect themselves against food scarcity. The problem came when technology and large-scale farming brought us into the agrarian revolution. People today eat because they want to, just because they fell like it, not necessarily because they need to.

The major problem with most of the modern diet is that it lacks a balanced supply of both macro and micronutrients. When you deprive your body of the nutrients it needs it will trigger a hunger stimulus to your brain and tell you to eat more. The body is trying to fix itself, so we have to make sure the food we eat is sending the right signals to our brains to keep our body healthy.

When you talk to many fitness advocates they will tell you to, just limit your calorie intake. By doing this your will take in less than you burn off and therefore you will lose weight. It sounds simple on the surface, but the major problem with this is that people get hungry. I mean let's be honest. If you are overweight and you are trying to cut calories you have to eat less. That takes a massive amount of will power and most people can't do it. That is why the majority of calorie counting diets fail miserably.

It's not your fault that you have failed at other diets.

The major benefits of the Paleo diet are that you get to eat things like unprocessed meats, vegetables, and fresh fruits; on top of that we can even add in some nuts. The special combination of foods you can eat will allow you to eat and fell full without eating too much or gorging yourself. Eating the right kinds of foods will trigger actions without your body allowing you to naturally lose weight without running for the nearest fast food joint. (I have been there before myself, I was so hungry I would grab anything and totally wreck any diet I was on, until Paleo.) Avoiding sugars and oils that contribute to gaining weight is one of the reasons that the Paleo diet is so successful.

What Is the Paleo Diet:

Understanding the Principles and Facts

If you are thinking about having a dieting program that really works in shedding off the fat deposit while improving your health level to the highest stage, you may want to consider about joining in the Paleo Diet. This kind of diet isn't something new; actually, but its popularity has just reached the peak level lately. You may be wondering what the Paleo diet is and what benefits you can achieve from it. In order to really understand about it, you need to take a look at the long history and progress in the making.

Also known as the Caveman diet or the Paleolithic diet

Also known as the Caveman diet or the Paleolithic diet, this kind of dieting program is based on the dieting concept during the ancient time - done by the cavemen. The cavemen diet theory itself is based on the researches and studies that most cavemen at that time were hunters. They are 'forced' to eat whatever they could find in the wild to survive. Whether they found veggies, fruits, or meat, they had to eat whatever provided for them. During the ancient time, there were no animals being domesticated; they were all hunted and eaten. There was no butter, cheese, milk, or other dairy products. This diet is mainly about consuming natural foods within their raw state, and that's how the program is implemented today.

Around 1970s, the theory about this dieting method has been discussed by Walter Voegtlin, but since there was also another poplar dieting program at that time - the Atkins diet - the Paleo dieting method is somehow forgotten and dismissed. But around 2005, this kind of dieting program started to appear again, thanks to Loren Cordain and the book of "The Paleo Diet for Athletes". At that time, lots of athletes were attracted to the book and they really implemented the methods after they had read the book. Afterwards, the Paleo diet started to get popular and it is considered as the new way in the dieting revolution.

However, there are several different concepts and understanding about how the program should be done. In one version, you are only allowed to eat the food within its raw state. For example, you are only allowed to eat animals that have been fed with natural grass only. However, in another version, you are allowed to consume dairy products. in short, it is quite difficult today to have Paleo diet that is truly on its raw and natural state. But some of the Paleo diet experts state that you can include and consume whatever you enjoy or comfortable eating, despite the basic and natural state. It is possible to have dairy products like cheese or milk, but keep in mind that they have high calories and they also have high level of fat. The most ideal foods that are similar to the cavemen diet are hard grains, legumes, and also potatoes.

It is important that you choose organic and natural raw food. You can also combine foods that have high level of carbs - like milk and potatoes - but you need to do the combination carefully as they have high level of calories. It would be better if you can combine veggies and fruits, along with proteins such as lean meat, beans, or nuts. If you are able to do these, you should feel great improvement in your health and fitness level.

Despite the benefit of having this kind of Paleo diet to help you lose weight, you need to remember that the main objective of the diet is not to lose weight, but it is all about life style changes. You can feel the benefits on longer terms and not within temporarily time range only. This kind of diet is claimed to be helpful to prevent serious and severe ailments such as diabetes, cardiovascular issues, high blood pressure, and so many more. It is also able to maintain proportional and ideal body weight while keeping the energy level stay intact. You should feel energized and strong on daily basis.

You need to consult your doctor first before doing this kind of diet. You need to make sure that your condition is okay and you are allowed to do this dieting program. It is also crucial to have your doctor monitor your progress and condition. Now that you know what the Paleo diet is, you can have discussion and consultation with your doctor about the best way to implement it.

The Many Benefits of The Paleo Diet

A Paleo diet is the 'cave mans' diet in short. Everything boiled, grilled and steamed. There are however a few exclusions including legumes, fatty meat, juices and sugary foods. All these should not be part of any Paleo diet. Rich fats and oil, lean meat, vegetables, nuts and fruits should be eaten in this case and prepared devoid of any processed fast and additives. The cave man solely survived on hunting and gathering. The premise is that they had to be lean enough to catch their next meals which meant that optimal health was not an option for you to eat.

These meals come with benefits that help you manage you weight among many other things. The best thing about a Paleo diet is that unlike many other diets, it is sustainable. You can stay on this diet the rest of your life and enjoy your meals immensely. The recipes and the food combinations will have your all your favorites only prepared differently. The meals need to be organically produced for them to pass this test. Any inorganically produced vegetables or fed animals will not qualify.

A strict Paleo diet will need to be researched well. Many people doing Paleo diets will miss it at some point due to the fat they have no idea how the food was created or brought up. Organic restaurants, grocers and butchers have now come up to help in his quest something that you can consider. Others have come up with their own organic gardens in the same quest and are making a difference in their lives. Here are some of the benefits of Paleo diets that should get you excited and going for this diet.

Fiber

Fiber is one of the main constituents of any pale diet. This is mostly found in vegetables. Fiber has a number of benefits in the body ranging from cleansing the system by sweeping dirt from the colon to helping in digestion. Fiber also eliminates any constipation, allows optimal absorption of water into the body and lowers the cholesterol levels. It also aids in lowering the risks of diabetes, coronary heart conditions and weight loss.

Weight Loss

The Paleo diet comes with lowered carbohydrate intake. The low nature of the diet in terms of starch is one of the benefits when it comes to attaining good weight loss. The fact that the meals are also devoid of fats eliminated the chances of any accumulation of the same in the system which is a great advantage.

Fibers and healthy fruits and vegetables will cleanse the body of any toxins that may cause damage t organs in the body like the liver and the kidney causing an increase in weight due to the slowing down of elimination of wastes. This increases metabolism and also helps the boy along in dealing with any wastes that might be closing the system.

Allergy Free Diet

The fact that the diet is casein and gluten free makes it ideal for everyone. These are major triggers when it comes to allergies related to food and nutrition. The will spark immunology responses that will trigger the body to react adversely to food and nay other inclusions. The absence of these keeps the body at peace and does not react to anything adversely.

Health Benefits In General

This diet comes with benefits that are related to the field of health in general. The fact that the diet can be sustained means that you will be picking a program that will last you a long time. One of the challenges when it comes to healthy dieting is the ability to stick to the program. The Paleo diet is a great diet that allows you to enjoy fruits, meats, fats and oil among many other foods as well.

You will enjoy a repressed appetite and an optimally functioning body with every part of the body being cleansed thanks to the diet. This diet is major risk reducer when it comes to arthritis, diabetes, many forms of cancer, goiter, high blood pressure, obesity, cardiovascular diseases and allergy related ailments. It is the perfect way to live worry free when it comes to you and your family.

A good Paleo diet needs to be well researched to ensure that it is correct. There are foods that are not allowed and those that are. Knowing this will keep you in a good position when it comes to your health goals through Paleo dieting.

Preparing For the Paleo Diet

How to Prepare for the Paleo Diet is certainly a question that many people who are considering this diet would like to know. After all, losing weight seems to be hit or miss with other diets out there, but the Paleo Diet seems to have had a lot of success and that is why it's so popular nowadays. So if you have decided to follow it, in the following paragraphs you will get to learn more about the right steps to take in this regard.

Preparation Mode

1. Setting a Start Date

First of all you'll need to download this calendar found at http://www.eat-real-food-Paleodietitian.com/support-files/calendar_tracking_tool_Paleo_challenge.pdf and then add in the date you want to get started with the diet.

It doesn't matter whether you want to start today, tomorrow or next week. But it's important you don't lose your motivation, so be sure you don't postpone it too many times.

2. Find Support

If you find support, then it will be easier for you to follow the diet. That is why you should try to maybe find a colleague, family member, spouse or friend who is willing to join you in hits challenge so you can support each other throughout the entire process. Don't worry if you have no one in your entourage, as you will find plenty of people on the internet who are willing to start the diet with you and encourage you on the way.

3. Take a Good Before Picture

Before you will start the diet, you will have to take a good picture of yourself, with the best pictures being the ones in which you wear little clothes. This is because you'll have something to compare yourself to after your twenty eight days dieting challenge.

You should also weigh yourself and take your body measurements as well.

Your doctor needs to be consulted for approval and you also need to have a complete blood work done (tests like blood pressure, CRP, LDL particle size, HDL, TG and blood sugars).

If you have any health problems or symptoms, then you should write them down.

4. Get Familiar with The Paleo Diet

Maybe you didn't really have time to learn all about the foods that you're going to eat during your Paleo challenge and if not, then you should take the time to learn about them. It's also a good idea to start looking for recipes you'll want to consider during your dieting challenge.

5. Clean Your Kitchen

If you have non-Paleo food in your kitchen, you'll have to get rid of all of it. It could be that you don't really want to just waste it, so you may try giving it to your colleagues, family members, friends or charitable organizations. However, think about it for a second? Do you really want your family members to eat unhealthy food?

You shouldn't feel bad about throwing away your food, because after all, this is a new beginning for you. A new lifestyle in which you'll only consider eating healthy foods to feel better and have a healthy BMI.

Action Mode

1. Start Stocking Up On Paleo Food

You should join a CSA program, visit the farmers market or just go grocery shopping.

It's recommended that you will bring the list of foods specific to your Paleo diet with you, so that you will not forget about the types of foods you should stock up on.

2. Stay Accountable And Keep Track

In order to track your progress you will have to use your calendar (each day you go through the Paleo diet needs to be crossed in the calendar, until you'll complete the entire twenty eight days challenge).

Bc surc you havc somconc to support you while considering the Paleo diet.

You may find it a good idea to actually keep a journal and write down everything you eat while you're following the Paleo diet. You may also take pictures of your meals and then upload them on a specialized website to keep track (one of them being PhotoCalorie dot com)

3. Hide the Scale

You may feel quite tempted to step on your scale before the twenty eight days challenge will be over, so that is why you should hide it. The reason behind this is the fact that the weight on the scale just doesn't tell you the full story and there are plenty of changes happening in your body that cannot be portrayed by the scale. Patience is the key in this regard.

It's important to focus on how you feel. That is why you should keep track of your symptoms, mood and energy levels in your daily journal.

4. Follow the Plan For Four Weeks

You should resist temptations as much as possible and avoid dairy, processed foods that contain sugar and \ or vegetable oils, legumes (like peanuts and soy) and of course, grains.

Your meals should be based on nuts, fruits, some tubers, but also healthy animal protein, healthy fats and vegetables.

Evaluation Mode

1. Now it's time to take your after picture

Use the same clothes you had when you took the before picture, weigh and also take your body measurements.

Do the blood work again and compare results.

Fill in the Paleo diet questionnaire and compare it to the one you filled in four weeks ago.

Assess the Results

Lastly, you should assess the results you got with this diet. If things got worse, you should ask yourself whether you were really serious about this challenge and if you cheated and why. Or it could be some of the foods contained ingredients you weren't allowed to have.

If things stayed the same, it could be that your body just needs a bit more time.

However, if things improved, then you can just stick to this diet and even tweak it to see how you'll feel and look after doing so.

Preparing for the Paleo diet is not something that's hard, but rather something you need to be involved in a bit more. After all, in 28 days you will basically manage to change your life, so it's definitely worth the effort!

What to Eat and What to Avoid On the Paleo Diet

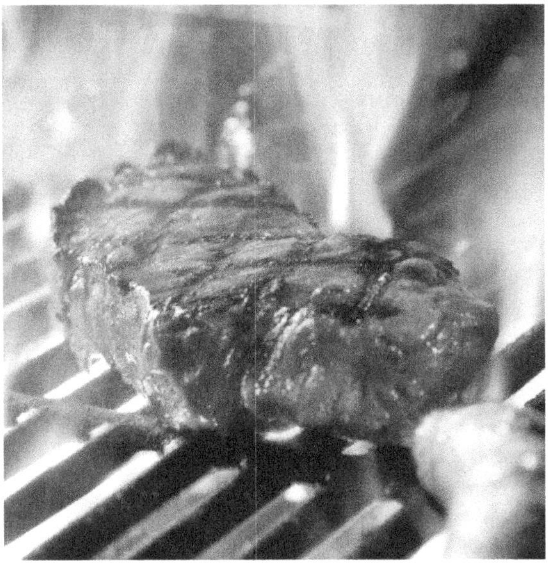

Download Your Complete Food List Here

http://just4u.co/o/paleobonus

A Paleo diet simply means eating foods that our ancestors did. The premise of this diet is that our forefathers were lean and healthy for a reason. They also lived longer when it came to surviving diseases related to diets. There is a reason why this was so. People have slowly shifted to aster ways of making food along with more harmful ways of doing the same.

Paleo diets are devoid of fats, cholesterol and other harmful food substances. One of the most common features of the Paleo diet is the preparation method. Foods were prepared through grilling or roasting, steaming and boiling. This kept hem healthy and fast enough to catch their prey. Here are some of the foods that you can eat and those that you need to avoid if you are looking to start a good Paleo diet.

Foods Allowed

The foods that are allowed for Paleo diet include Meats, vegetables, oils and fats, nuts and fruits. The Paleo meats that are allowed in this list will include meat from herbivores, birds and fish. These meats will need to be prepared in a certain way for them to be considered Paleo. The meat will either need to be boiled or grilled. All the fat in the meat also needs to be eliminated. The meat also had to be organic for it to qualify as Paleo.

The diet will also need vegetables. These should be eaten raw or boiled. They include lettuce, cabbage, cauliflower, kales, celery and many more. They should never be overcooked or fried in any situation. Oil and fats from fish are part of the Paleo diet. These are rich in omega 3 components among many other benefits which are good for the body. These will also not cause any harmful deposits in the body. Animal fats are not allowed into the meals keeping everything lean.

Nuts and fruits are a great source of vitamins and beneficial fats. These are either roasted or eaten raw.

Foods Not Allowed

There are also foods that are not allowed in a Paleo diet. These include Dairy products like cheese, milk and butter. Soft drinks like soda and processed juices are an absolute 'No' in the diet too. One should keep clear of legumes like beans and grains, fatty meats, salty foods, starchy vegetables, snacks, sweets and energy drinks.

All these have the side effect of adding weight and also increasing the cholesterol levels in the body. Their fats and components take the body long to process and in some cases will cause a problem in the normal functioning leading to constipation, bloating and indigestion.

A Paleo diet unlike many other diets in the market today can be sustained over a long time which is a good thing. One of the biggest issues that come with dieting is that people will resume habits that will cause a rebound in weight gain. Paleo diets can be managed over a long time and even become a lifestyle.

Common Mistakes to Avoid On the Paleo Diet

Most of the mistakes that people do in Paleo Diet are caused by ignorance and lack of proper understanding on how the diet works. Some of the common mistakes to avoid on the Paleo diet are:

Mistake #1

1. Trying To Completely Eliminate Intake Of Fats From Their Diet.

Since Paleo diet's function is to control your weight, most of the people try to eliminate any traces of fat from their food so as to prevent themselves from gaining excess weight. This is not the actual solution to losing weight. Fats help in food digestion and absorption of some important nutrients in the body. It is necessary to include some amount of fat in your diet as it goes a long way in boosting your health needs. This avoids harming your body.

Mistake #2

2. People Try To Make Everything In The Paleo Diet In Every Meal.

This causes undue pressure and stress to the individuals. It causes unnecessary craving for the foods and may lead to a kind of threat in the functioning of your body. The actual problem is that a lot of people fluctuate between extremes, in actual fact- you ought to have little treats during different times of the day as long as it doesn't end up becoming the mainstay in all your diets. This is because the primary focus of the diet is to incline on eating plenty of natural vegetables and meat.

Mistake #3

3. Eating More Nuts Than Are Recommended.

As nuts play a crucial part of the Paleo diet, people often make the mistake of eating as many nuts as they can. The truth of the matter is that the excess nuts do not help you in losing weight. Excessive consumption of the nuts will actual hinder the weight reduction process and actually make you add more weight.

Mistake #4

4. People Also Have The Wrong Notion About Losing Weight. It Leads To People Skipping Necessary Meals Thus Leading To Binges.

Most of the people tend to deprive their bodies the right quantity of nutrients they require when they eating less so as to reduce weight gain. This is a wrong way of losing weight. Binging in your diets only results to metabolisms going haywire thus affecting you negatively. The way forward is to regular eat meals but at lesser promotions.

Mistake #5

5. Expect To Lose Weight In A Short Time Frame Work.

Most people are often disappointed after eating the Paleo diet for a week and it seems not to have worked. You should be aware that the diet is not a term process where you expect to see its effects in a week. It is a lifelong process that allows you to achieve your desired weight. Becoming too ambitious will result to failure of the process and you will not have the patience to go along with the diet and continue following it. If you are not a patient person, this is not the right place to be!

Mistake #6

6. Trying To Eat Junk Food Paleo.

It is does not make sense trying to replace junk foods with Paleo equivalents. Even thou there are packaged food with Paleo labels, these foods cannot be compared to the actual homemade Paleo diet as they may not contain the required ingredients.

In order to avoid such common mistakes in the Paleo diet, people have to be a little more careful in understanding the diet completely so as to avoid such small mistakes.

Mistake #7

7. Keeping An Open Mind to Change

You have to have the right mindset to really want to make a change in your life. Most times people look for a diet because of a health problem. But, you have to make the diet not just a diet, but a way of life. Think about it. A diet is something someone does to drop some quick weight, but you need a life change, a new way of living.

So if you don't take away anything else from this book, remember this. You need to REALLY want to make a positive change in your life. This is not a diet, it is a way of life for you to be healthy and potentially avoid further health complications.

Quick Reminder if You Missed It
Customer Only Bonus

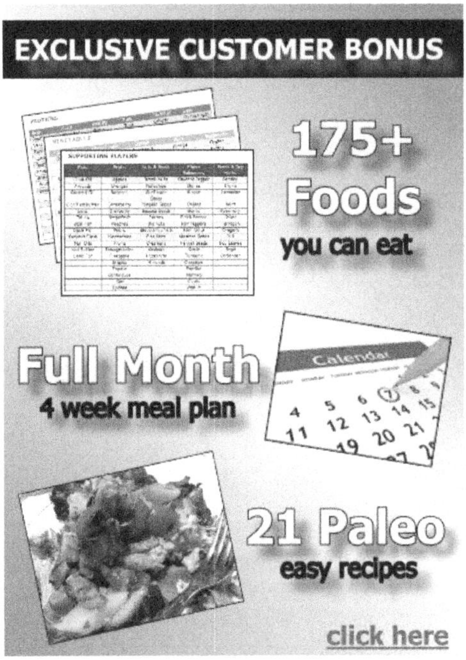

You can also get the customer appreciation bonus here:

http://just4u.co/o/paleobonus